CONQUER CHRONIC PAIN!
SEVEN PRINCIPLES THAT SHOW YOU HOW

CONQUER CHRONIC PAIN!
SEVEN PRINCIPLES THAT SHOW YOU HOW

BY TODD W. USSERY, MD
BOARD-CERTIFIED PAIN-MANGEMENT PHYSICIAN

Conquer Chronic Pain!/Todd W. Ussery --1st ed.

ISBN: 9781704344324

Illustrations by Kierston Vande Kraats (kenriots.carbonmade.com)

Editing and book design by Kevin Miller (www.kevinmillerxi.com)

DEDICATION

For Christine, my fellow conqueror.

Disclaimer

This book details the author's personal experiences with and opinions about chronic pain management. This book does not make the author your healthcare provider. If you are a patient of the author, this book is not part of his clinical medical practice and does not constitute clinical advice to you.

The author and publisher are providing this book and its contents on an "as is" basis and make no representations or warranties of any kind with respect to this book or its contents. Although the intent is to provide accurate information, the author and publisher disclaim all such representations and warranties, including for example warranties of merchantability and healthcare for a particular purpose. In addition, the author and publisher do not represent or warrant that the information accessible via this book is accurate, complete or current. The statements made about products and services have not been evaluated by the U.S. Food and Drug Administration. They are not intended to diagnose, treat, cure, or prevent any condition or disease. Please consult with your own physician or healthcare specialist regarding the suggestions and recommendations made in this book. Except as specifically stated in this book, neither the author or publisher, nor any authors, contributors, or other representatives will be liable for damages arising out of or in connection with the use of this book.

This is a comprehensive limitation of liability that applies to all damages of any kind, including (without limitation) compensatory; direct, indirect or consequential damages; loss of data, income or profit; loss of or damage to property and claims of third parties. You understand that this book is not intended as a substitute for consultation with a licensed healthcare practitioner, such as your physician. Before you begin any healthcare program, or change your lifestyle in any way, you will consult your physician or another licensed healthcare practitioner to ensure that you are in good health and that the examples contained in this book will not harm you.

This book provides content related to physical and/or mental health issues. As such, use of this book implies your acceptance of this disclaimer.

Contents

Introduction

We were just getting out of a morning service at church when a woman named Julia approached me in the lobby.[1] "Hi, Dr. Todd. Good to see you. Are you doing well?"

"I sure am," I replied. "You're looking good today too. I guess last week's epidural steroid got rid of that flare-up."

She smiled. "By the next day, I was walking great again. Thanks so much for fitting me in on short notice.

"By the way, my brother, Carlos, is visiting me this week. He lives about six hours away. He hurt his back three months ago at work and has been on light duty since then. I told him how the epidurals helped me, so he went to a physician who did them. They did an MRI that showed a bulging disk, which confirmed where the pain was coming from, so they did three epidurals."

"I hope they helped," I said.

"Well, no they didn't," she replied, shaking her head. "Maybe you do them better? Anyway, can he set up an appointment with you to see him and do another epidural?"

I agreed to see Carlos later that week, and then Julia and I said our goodbyes.

When I met with Carlos, he expressed his frustration. "I was moving a box when I felt a little pop on one side. I felt a bit of pain right away but not too bad. The next day the pain was excruciating, starting in my back and radiating down the side of my leg almost to the knee. It hurt to stand and walk."

"How is it now?" I asked. He seemed uncomfortable, especially getting out of a chair or when he started to walk.

1 Names, some details, and locations have been changed to maintain privacy in this and all references to patient's stories.

"It's better than that first week, but it has never gone away. The back pain is the worst. Every time I try to do my full job, it flares up. The next day I can hardly walk. I'm concerned I won't be able to keep my job if it doesn't clear up soon."

"Do you have numbness below the knee or weakness in the affected leg?" I asked, a question that would help me determine the source of pain.

"No numbness. My leg gives out on me sometimes, but I catch myself. The doctor that I saw ordered an MRI, which showed a herniated disk on the side of the pain. He did three epidural steroid injections three weeks apart. They helped a few days each but didn't last."

I did an exam on Carlos that showed normal reflexes in his legs and no weakness. I looked at the MRI he had brought. It showed a herniation on the side of the painful leg among other disk herniations and signs of degeneration common for his age throughout the spine.

"I think it's unlikely that the disc herniation is causing your pain," I said. "Instead, I think you probably have an inflamed joint in your low back. An epidural would not give lasting relief to the joint since it was meant to treat the nerve root."

Carlos was shocked. "Why did the MRI show a herniated disk then? And why did the doctor say the radiating pain down my leg showed it was from the nerve root?"

"You don't have the symptoms or signs of a true radicular pain, which would involve pain in a narrow band going below the knee toward the foot, indicating the problem was from an inflamed nerve root," I replied. "The MRI showed a herniated disk on that side but also other herniations and degeneration. The MRI cannot show pain. Most structural problems that show up on the image do not cause any pain at all."

As I spoke, I saw his disappointment grow, so I quickly added some encouragement. "We can get you in for a ten-minute procedure tomorrow under X-ray to show us the actual pain source. If we confirm that the pain is coming from the joint, we can treat it fairly simply."

I performed a diagnostic block with local anesthetic to the medial branch nerve that carried pain from the facet joint of the low back. It and a confirmatory diagnostic block revealed the facet joint to be the source of his pain. Using a non-surgical radiofrequency probe, I deadened the nerve, leaving him with minimal pain. He went back to work with full duties within a couple of weeks.

A month later I saw Julia at church again. "How's your brother?" I asked.

"He's doing great! He even went back to playing softball in his local league," she said, beaming. Then her brow furrowed. "Why do you think his first doctor made the mistake about his true diagnosis?"

"He made the diagnosis overly influenced by the MRI. He saw abnormalities that could cause back pain and jumped to the conclusion that it was the pain source. The same thing happens time and again. In fact, a mistake in the pain diagnosis is neither unusual nor considered erroneous." We parted ways at the front of the church, but my mind stayed on the problem of treating pain.

Using Wisdom to Treat Chronic Pain

Treatment of pain can be done better! With the help of inexpensive, low-risk testing techniques that are well established and medically proven to establish a pain diagnosis that accurately identifies the source of pain, ineffective and expensive procedures can be drastically curtailed. Once a diagnosis is made, procedures can be sorted by effectiveness and risk, thus reducing unwanted long-term side effects. Providers have a responsibility to their patients to know the most effective and lowest-risk method of treating the condition before them, whether they can perform the treatment themselves or not.

Pain management involves more than procedures though. Most of the disability brought on by chronic pain is preventable. Muscles in the back that go unused for years become shortened, weak, and painful, though they did not sustain the primary injury. Fears and distorted beliefs prevent sufferers from keeping these muscles strong and supple.

A good pain-management plan will head off loss of function and provide a way to restore what has been needlessly lost. The type of foods you eat, your activity level, and whether you smoke or use alcohol or drugs have a direct effect on daily pain levels and level of function.

This book is for anyone with chronic pain who wants a guide to help them choose the right path of treatment, whether you are new to the confusing world of pain management or have learned too many lessons the hard way and would welcome some good advice. I will teach you seven universal and critical principles applied to the treatment of chronic pain. They are ordered in such a way as to follow the progression of a chronic pain patient from selecting a pain-management provider to expanding to a team of surgeons, therapists, and counselors, as needed, and finally to centering on the development of the resilience needed to live contentedly and prosper in whatever state you find yourself after all that can be done has been or is currently being done.

I applaud you for reading this far. It already puts you ahead of 99 percent of new pain-management patients. You are where you need to be to start a journey of victory and wisdom. If you want, take a moment to skip ahead to the last chapter to discover where the seven principles come from. If not, turn the page and take the first step toward overcoming your chronic pain.

The Principle of Individuality

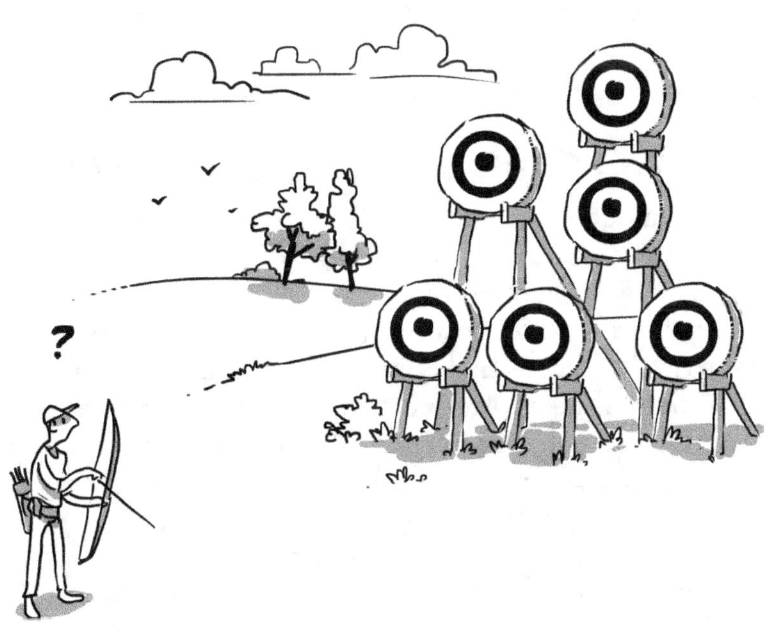

Each patient has a unique identity that requires an individual plan.

Application to pain management: You must get a pain diagnosis. To make a treatment plan, you must know the precise source of your pain.

Versions of Carlos's story, as recounted in the introduction, take place repeatedly in the lives of those suffering from chronic pain. His doctor did not get an accurate pain diagnosis, which led to a useless procedure. The mistake was based on the findings of an MRI of the low back. While Carlos had had X-rays in the past, X-rays cannot show a herniated disk. This was the first MRI ever done on his back and it showed a herniated disk, so the doctor assumed the disk was causing the pain.

Other findings did not confirm the doctor's assumption. The examination of the back was not diagnostic for nerve root pain. Carlos had deep radiating pain down the leg but he had worse pain above the knee and no loss of reflexes (see Table 1, number 5, at the end of this chapter). Pain from a nerve root won't always have all these symptoms and signs, but without such clear-cut evidence, a more comprehensive workup is needed to find the actual source of pain (as seen in Figure 1). The prevalence of facet joint pain may be up to 41 percent. The prevalence of sacroiliac joint pain is up to 25 percent. Epidural steroids are not a first-line treatment for either of these sources of pain. In Carlos's case, the source of pain was a facet joint.

You Can't See Pain on an MRI

A little while ago, I sat waiting to hear an academic pain-management physician, an expert in pain source diagnosis. The room was packed for his lecture, a reflection of his reputation.

"Overreliance on MRIs causes many needless and possibly harmful back surgeries," he said. "That is an astonishing fact. The more astonishing fact is that this takes place even though MRI's unreliability in establishing a pain source has been known for decades but still continues. As late as 2019, experts warned that reliance on imaging in the diagnosis of the pain source leads directly to failed procedures."

He brought up some statistics of findings on MRIs of volunteers with no pain. "Structural abnormalities of the spine are present in all patients. By their forties most people without any back pain will have a number of abnormalities on an MRI that would be considered surgical. When those patients have their first MRI, one often cannot differentiate which of many abnormalities is the pain source. Removing or correcting spinal abnormalities found on imaging may fail to cure pain and may even worsen it."

He paused and looked at the group. "So what is the answer to such a diagnostic dilemma?"

What does the MRI of someone with no pain look like?

In a study of MRI results of a volunteer population, 83 percent had moderate to severe disc desiccation of one or more disk (often called a black disc), 64 percent had one or more bulging discs, 56 percent had loss of disc height, 32 percent had at least one disc protrusion, and 6 percent had one or more disc extrusions. None of them had pain.

"An accurate diagnosis (finding the true pain source) is necessary for effective treatment and to prevent needless surgeries. While there is no universally accepted gold standard for spine pain diagnosis, local anesthetic blocks, properly performed, are by far the closest method to a finding the true source of pain. Attempting to use the description of the pain, physical exams, imaging (often an MRI), and nerve conduction studies in non-radicular back pain identifies the precise cause of pain in only 15 percent of patients. However, controlled diagnostic nerve blocks bring that percentage up to 85 percent."

Medial Branch Blocks and Radiofrequency Ablations

The joints in the back (the ones you hear when you "crack your back") are generally referred to as facet joints. These joints get arthritis (degeneration) in them like other joints in the body from a combination of aging, trauma, and overloading. They are the most common cause of back pain when the back pain is worse than leg pain. Degeneration in these joints is not treated directly by surgery. Diagnosis of a painful facet joint is done by placing a local anesthetic (like lidocaine) over the medial branch nerve that carries the pain from the joint. If that stops or almost stops the pain, then the pain is most likely coming from the joint. Currently, the treatment for a painful joint is ablation of the medial branch nerve using a special radiofrequency probe that heats it up.

Here are my recommendations for getting an accurate pain diagnosis:
- When back pain is worse than leg pain, numbness does not strictly follow the coverage of the nerve (the dermatome), or no reflexes are lost, do not assume the pain is caused by impingement on the nerve root. Get further testing.

- Insist on testing from your new pain-management physician, even if you have held a diagnosis for years, unless the original diagnosis was made using diagnostic blocks.

- Get a pain diagnosis for any new type of pain or pain in a new area that arises even when already getting treatment, even if the treatment helps alleviate it.

- Remember, MRI is a great tool to see destruction of the spine, but you can't see pain on an MRI.

Common Causes of Low Back Pain
(with percentage of total causes)

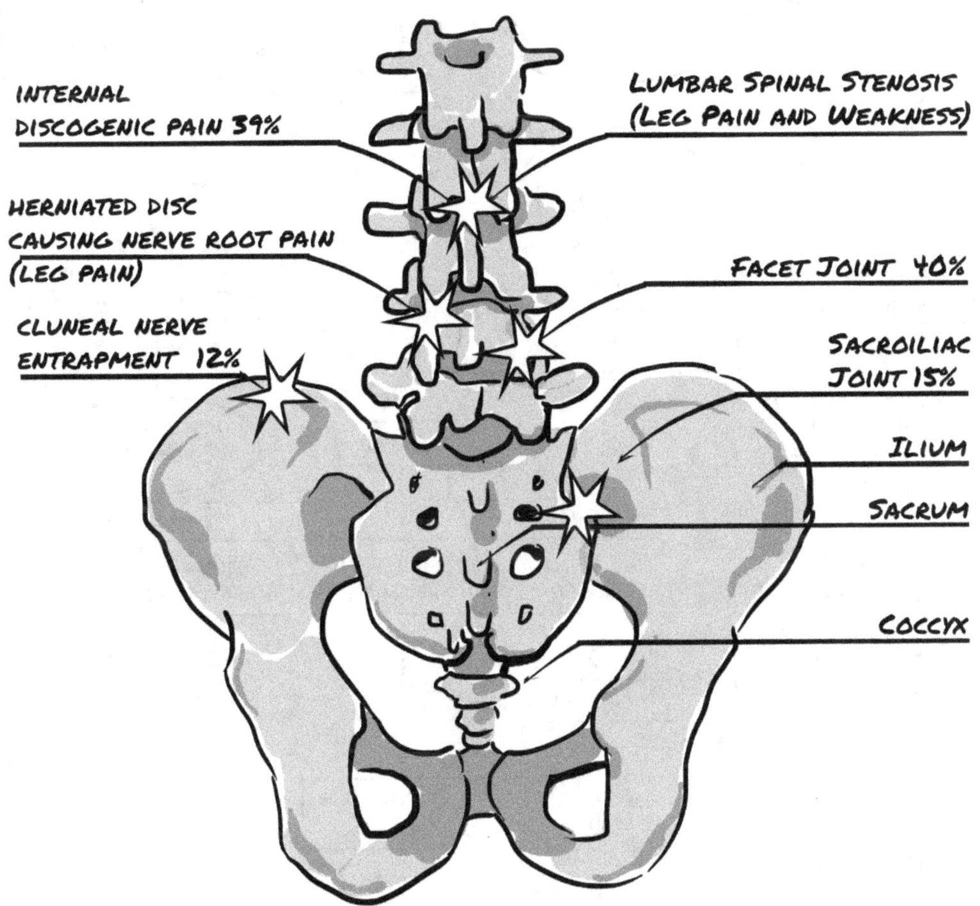

Chronic Low Back Pain Algorithm

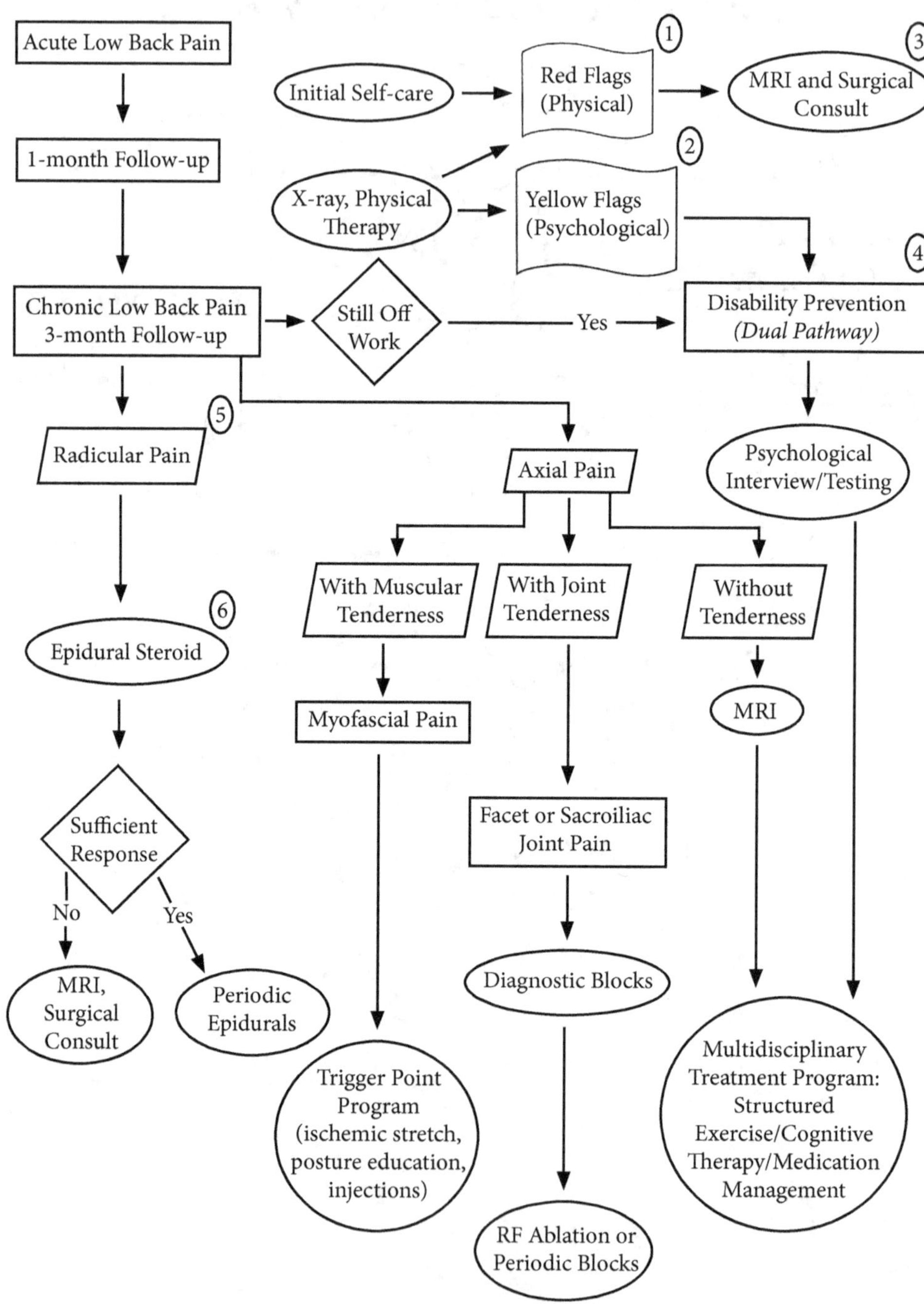

Table 1:
Key to Chronic Low Back Pain Algorithm

1. Red flags are potential emergencies requiring surgery.

2. Yellow flags are psychological or social risk factors for long-term disability and work loss.

3. In the absence of red flags, an MRI is not helpful before many low-risk treatments. Overall, the MRI poorly correlates with the pain source.

4. Eighty-five percent of patients are back to work within three months. The race to prevent long-term disability begins when recovery stalls or yellow flags are identified.

5. For lower-limb pain, referred pain is much more common than true radiculopathy. All characteristics listed may not be present.

	Radicular Pain (Nerve Root)	**Referred Pain**
Nature of Pain	Shooting, electrical	Dull, aching, pressure
Location	Below knee > above knee Narrow band of pain Deep and superficial pain	Above knee > below knee Wide band, indistinct boundaries Deep pain only
Neurological	May have weakness/reduced reflexes/dense numbness	Normal neurologically/may have mild numbness

6. A transforaminal approach to lumbar epidurals targets the nerve root at a specific side and level.

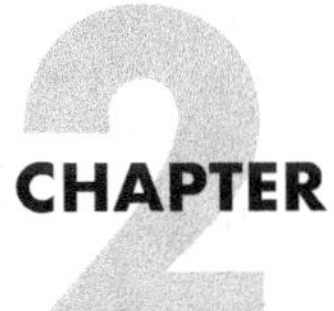

The Principle of Leadership

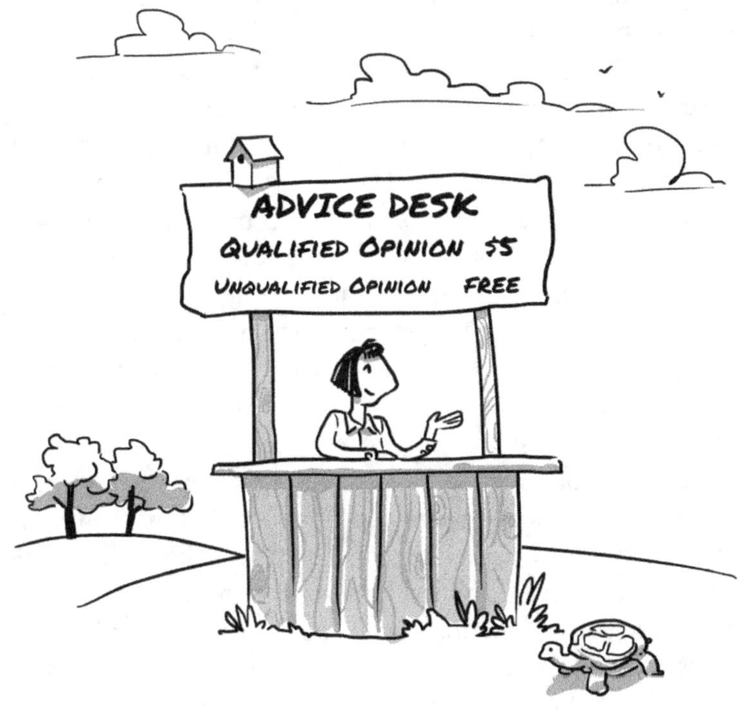

Those who serve us have unique spheres of responsibility.

Application to pain management: Providers are responsible to be knowledge-able in their area of expertise and to seek consultation where they are not.

When I met Bill in the examination room, he was anxious. "I want to know if there is any procedure that could be done to keep me working."

I asked him how his pain started.

"I developed neck pain in my mid-thirties," he said. "Over the next ten years, I tried every possible treatment available. I had many series of physical therapy and steroid injections. Eventually, I had a cervical fusion. I'm taking a non-steroidal, an antidepressant, and I started chronic opioid treatment five years ago. I continued to work full time."

"That's admirable," I said.

"Yeah, I felt that my life was a delicate balance between rest and medications to continue to work to maintain myself and my family. It was worth it though."

He looked down. "What happened next disrupted that balance. When my physician retired and turned his practice over to a new partner, I thought nothing of it. Little did I know the crisis it would bring to my life. The new physician sat me down in his office for a talk. 'The opioids you're taking are very addictive,' he said, 'and studies have shown that long-term opioids are ineffective, so I'm going to wean you off them.' I was scared, but I followed his advice. I started missing work because of pain, and my job was in jeopardy for the first time in five years. I finally convinced my new physician to send me to pain management to see if anything could be done to keep me from going on disability."

After getting some more details and doing a thorough exam, I sat down with Bill. "We can test over the next few months for a procedure that will help," I said, "but I know how to get you back to where you were before within a week."

He looked at me in surprise. "How?"

"By putting you back on opioids," I replied. "You were taking a moderate dose of hydrocodone for years and doing well. You showed no sign of addiction or misuse. We know it works for you with minimal side effects. You have proven yourself low risk, and the system used to monitor you will help provide early detection if you start to drift toward misuse."

Bill's eyes welled up as he began to see hope of keeping his job. We talked more about the risks of opioids and the protocols my clinic had in place to decrease those risks. I called his primary-care doctor and discussed my recommendations with him. He agreed when he heard the meticulous care my clinic took in monitoring patients on opioids. Bill went back to his former level of performance and retired many years later.

The Opioid Crisis and Chronic Pain

Make no mistake, opioids are dangerous drugs. The three main risks are overdose, addiction, and divergence (the giving or selling of one's prescribed drugs to others). In response to a national increase in overdoses from prescription opioids, coined the "opioid crisis," state and national regulatory bodies acted to drastically reduce their supply across the board. Overall prescriptions of opioids in the nation fell by well over half between 2012 and 2017. Opioid deaths from prescription opioids increased little between 2009 and 2017, but deaths related to synthetic narcotics, predominately fentanyl, increased 898 percent. Government agencies and state medical societies were successful in cutting the supply of prescription drugs but not the number of prescription opioid deaths. Unfortunately, the total opioid death rate continued to rise because abusers found ready alternate, illegal sources.

Another less-publicized crisis arose directly from the efforts to quell the opioid crisis, which involved existing chronic pain patients. Fearing government censure, too many providers throughout the country curtailed the dose or completely cut off long-term opioid prescriptions. Many patients who kept a fragile balance of productivity in their lives became practically bedridden. This travesty is still being sorted out as these patients are transferred to pain clinics.

As laws have become more arduous for physicians prescribing long-term opioids, more and more primary care doctors are sending the patients to whom they were formerly prescribing opioids to pain-management clinics. Of patients presenting to pain clinics with chronic pain, 94 percent are already taking chronic opioids. In general, pain-management providers continue patients on opioids much more often than they initiate them.

Using Opioids Wisely

Changes in prescribing should rely on good scientific evidence and take individual patients' circumstances to account. The risks of any medication must be weighed against the benefits. I have declined to order opioids to countless new patients because their past actions place them at too high a risk of misuse, and I have stopped prescribing many who have failed to follow the rules once they started. This process is factual and non-judgmental. Except when they have lied to me, I usually continue to treat those patients with lower-risk medications.

Getting Off Opioids

So far, no low-risk wonder drug relieves pain like opioids do. Opioids are still unique among medications in providing pain relief for severe neuropathic and non-neuropathic pain. Proper titration (concentration of the drug) can avoid excessive sedation, the drug's most dangerous side effect. Almost all overdoses involve misuse.

If your pain is mild to moderate, you may get off opioids with the wise use of adjunctive medications and/or periodic office procedures. A small number of patients with severe nerve-related pain can be treated with just adjunctive drugs. However, the only current alternatives to opioids for most severe chronic pain conditions are procedures that remove or destroy painful tissue or implantable devices that modulate the nerves carrying the painful responses.

Not All Pain-management Clinics Are the Same

A full-spectrum pain-management clinic is effective in identifying what treatment will work for you. Two extremes can make a pain clinic less effective. The first is a clinic that concentrates on opioids and a few other prescriptions with little face-to-face time with patients, usually neglecting the emotional or social aspects of a patient's condition. Such providers only do quick office procedures. In contrast, procedures that can replace some or all the opioids a patient is taking are usually done in a surgery center or hospital. A physician who does not do these state-of-the-art procedures will often not even mention them.

The second extreme is the "interventional only" physician who provides procedures but not medication. This is a legitimate business decision for the physician, but patients must find another provider to continue their medication management.

Overall, you are more likely to get comprehensive treatment from a provider who offers a comprehensive approach rather than trying to patch together multiple providers, though for mild to moderate chronic pain, this may not be an issue.

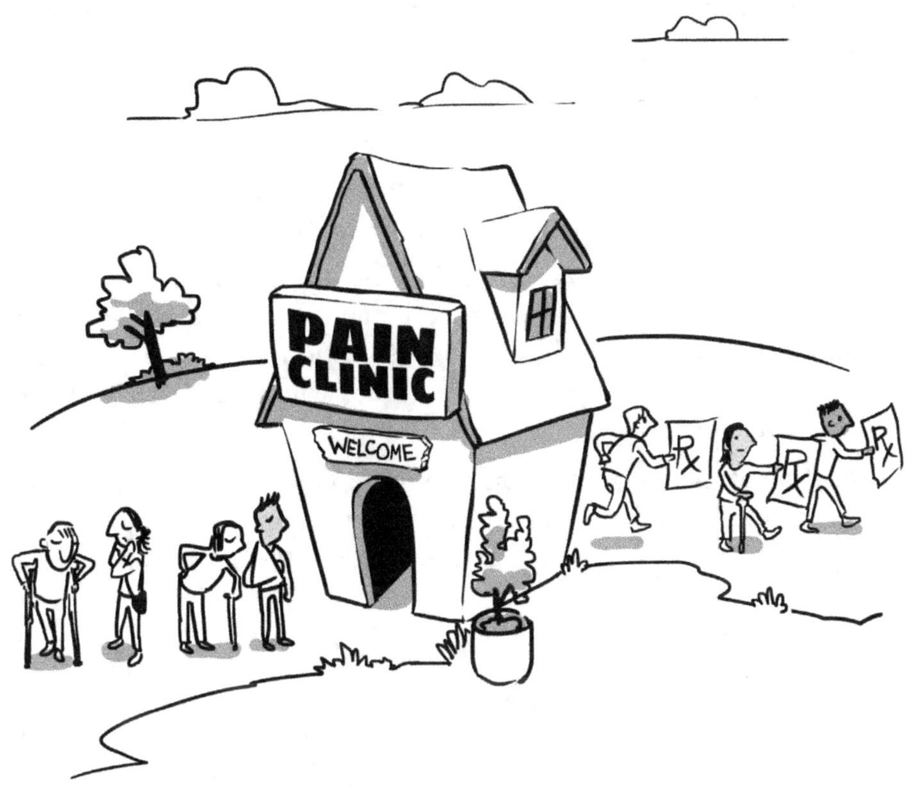

Getting a Second Opinion

Every provider has the right to decide what he or she will prescribe, but in giving advice in controversial areas, I believe providers should stay close to their area of expertise. I stay in my lane, so to speak. "First do no harm" is an axiom long held foundational in modern medicine, whether doing procedures, giving medications, or dispensing advice. For example, if a patient asks me if I would recommend a surgery that he or she has been offered, I give the patient the success rate of that surgery just for the relief of pain, if such information is available. If the reason for the surgery involves instability or conditions other than pain, I defer. For procedures that carry anything above a low risk (most of these are surgeries), I usually recommend a second opinion with another physician who does the same type of case who is not related to or in business with the physician who would do the procedure. A nearby town often provides enough distance if your town is small. Get a referral from the first physician, so you receive an official opinion in writing, not casual advice.

My recommendations for choosing a pain-management provider are:

- If you have moderate to severe chronic pain, get established with a pain physician.

- Choose a pain-management physician who does medication management and procedures. Medications should include opioids as an option, even if you don't need them at this point.

- If you have moderate to severe pain, a pain clinic that only does procedures in the office is unlikely to be able to decrease your opioid using these office procedures and medications. If decreasing opioid use is one of your goals, find a provider who does state-of-the-art procedures in a surgery center or hospital.

- Don't be afraid to get a second opinion. Doctors are used to being questioned nowadays. Definitely get one for any procedure that is higher than low risk and possibly before starting chronic opioid treatment.

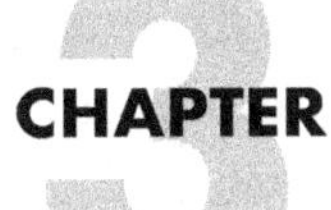

The Principle of Unity and Union

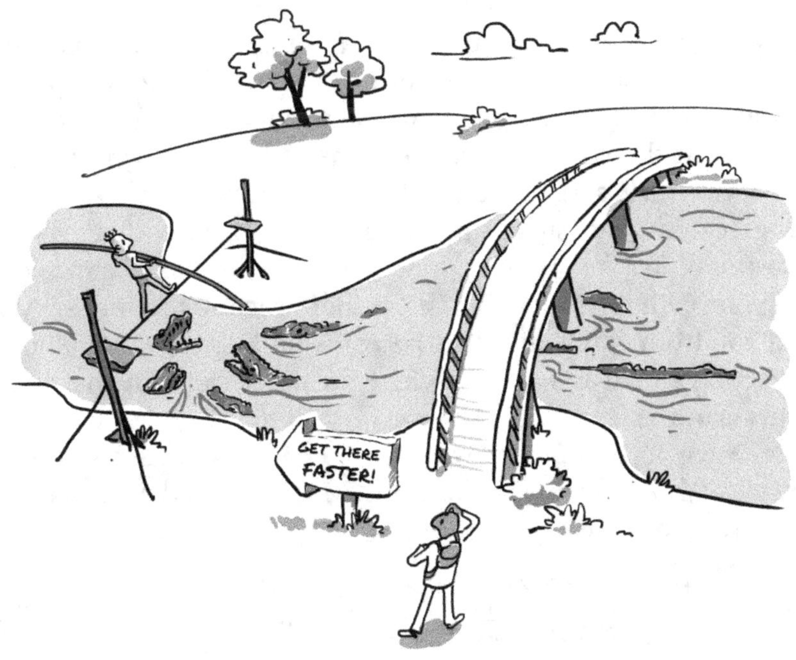

Parts work together when they are united in principle.

Application to pain management: All your providers should routinely follow the concept of graduated risk.

oe came to me after being sent by his surgeon, a respected physician and a good friend of mine, for an initial consult.

"I'm an engineer. I've always been a hard worker. Five years ago I reached down to pick up a dropped tool and was bent over by excruciating back and left-leg pain. I did a month of physical therapy, which helped but not enough," he told me. "The surgeon who sent me here examined me, ordered an MRI, and diagnosed me as having radiculopathy due to a disc herniation on the left side. I had a relatively simple laminectomy spine surgery that removed some disc material and bone, and I was back to full duty at work as good as new in a few weeks."

"That's a great surgery," I said.

He nodded. "Yeah, it was, but six weeks ago it happened again. I got the same pain, this time on the right side. I went back to the same surgeon. He did another MRI, which showed the leftover disk was touching the nerve."

"So the same surgeon who did a good job could do the other side, right?" I asked.

He shrugged. "That's the thing. Because of the bone removed previously, the next surgery would need to include a fusion to maintain structural strength. I've known coworkers who've had fusions, and I'm nervous about the risks involved and the time off from work that I'll need to recover. He sent me to you to discuss options."

"I agree with your surgeon," I assured Joe. "I have lower-risk treatments with almost no recovery time that have the same chance of alleviating your pain. The nice thing is, if they aren't successful, they won't prevent you from going ahead with the fusion. I can do an epidural steroid injection aimed at the space where the nerve exits. The herniation is likely to shrink over time."

After a few injections, Joe was back to work. He had two more over the next year. After a couple of years, an MRI showed the herniation had shrunk away from the nerve.

Transforaminal and Translaminar
Epidural Steroid Injections

One of the most commonly used pain procedures is the epidural steroid injection. The epidural space lies between the tough covering over the spinal fluid and the ligaments attached to the bones of the spine. Medicine in this space migrates to the spinal cord and to the spinal roots that exit the spine to become nerves. Steroids decrease production of pain chemicals and decrease swelling. Many times the decrease in swelling is enough to stop the cause of the pain, though a flare-up can repeat the cycle of pain and swelling. In that case, another epidural could stop it again.

Transforaminal epidurals are the most focused method of placing medication where it is most needed. The thin needle is inserted through the foramen, the bony exit for the nerve root most affected, and the steroid is made available where disks and ligaments are most likely to press against nerve tissue. The other approach is between the lamina, the back struts of the spine. This technique is less specific but can be very helpful therapeutically.

Always Start with Low-risk Procedures

Joe's initial surgery, a simple laminectomy, had low risk, high effectiveness, and moderate cost (see Table 2). In contrast, the second surgery, involving a fusion, had moderate effectiveness, moderate risk, and high cost. Even if insurance covered most of the expense, the cost to Joe in recovery time spent off work and reduced duty (many times around six months to a year) was significant. In addition, the procedure places stress on the spinal disks and joints above and below the fusion, causing them to become painful and often requiring another fusion a few years later!

He chose to try an epidural steroid treatment because its effectiveness is also moderate, but the long-term risk and the cost are low. Recovery from an epidural is a few days at most, usually just one day, and the procedure does not lead to breakdown of other segments over the long term, like the surgical fusion. A number of patients get a few epidurals with complete resolution of all pain. In some cases epidural steroids don't give sufficient pain relief, perhaps because of bony impingement or the progress of disk shrinking is too slow. In these cases the laminectomy is a good early treatment with high effectiveness, low risk, and moderate cost.

In most cases epidural steroids, in the absence of other urgent issues, should be tried before surgery. In cases of low back pain without neurologic complications, instability, or other critical issues, a lumbar fusion should be considered only after low-risk procedures have failed or been ruled out.

Table 2

Pain Procedure	Effectiveness	Risk	Cost
Radiofrequency Ablation Medial Branch Lumbar	Moderate	Low	Low
Lumbar Laminectomy	High	Low	Moderate
Lumbar Fusion Surgery	Moderate	Moderate	High
Epidural Steroid Injection	Moderate	Low	Low
Spinal Cord Stimulator after Trial	High	Low	Moderate
Peripheral Nerve Stimulator after Trial	High	Low	Moderate
Radiofrequency Ablation Medial Branch Cervical	Moderate	Low	Low
Diagnostic Medial Branch Blocks – All Levels	High	Low	Low
Peripheral Nerve Blocks for Long-term Pain	Moderate	Low	Low
Peripheral Joint Injections for Long-term Pain	Moderate	Low	Low
PRP Injections to Joints, Ligaments, and Tendons	Moderate	Low	High
Chronic Opioid Management	Moderate	Moderate	Low
Diagnostic Peripheral Nerve Blocks	High	Low	Low

Joe made his decision by weighing the risks and the benefits. His surgeon and I had the same philosophy of treatment, so we were able to come up with a wisely thought out plan. We both adhered to the concept of graduated risk, comparing each treatment's effectiveness, risk, and cost, and then ordering the low-risk procedures first.

One should not fall into the deception that skipping less-risky treatments is the same as going for a cure. Increase in risk does not correlate with greater effectiveness. Graduated risk is an established standard of care in modern medicine. If a physician advises jumping straight to a higher-risk option, he or she should be able to justify this decision to the patient and another physician in the same field.

My recommendations for choosing procedures according to the concept of graduated risk:

- Make sure you know the options for treatment and that you start with effective but low-risk before moderate- or high-risk interventions

- Except in an emergency, get a second opinion for any moderate- or high-risk procedures

The Principle of Sowing and Reaping

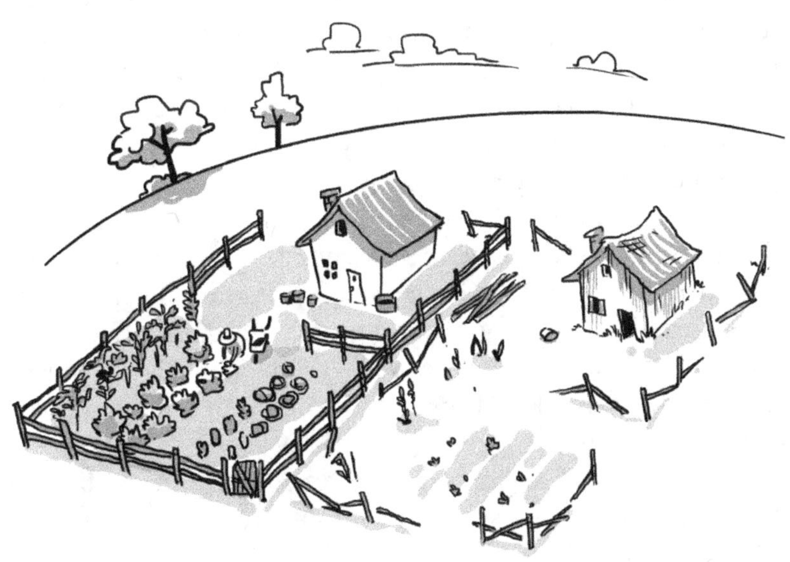

The actions you take each day will add up to success or failure.

Application to pain management: Brief and consistent exercise and stretching produce significant long-lasting rewards.

Physical therapy doesn't work for me. I tried it once, and I hurt worse than before I started. I do stretching and exercise at home, the same as at physical therapy. Besides, I'm busy watching my grandchildren, and I get plenty of exercise doing that," Ellen declared the first time I met her. "I take four oxycodone a day. I want to stick with that."

But was she really OK?

She was unable to shop alone because of chronic pain in her shoulders when her arms were raised. Taking a can off the shelf had become excruciating. When she pushed her limits, she paid for it the next day with increased pain and stiffness. In addition, her pain had become worse over time and spread, starting with an original injury in her shoulders but now extending into her back on both sides.

I knew what I had to say, but I also realized I was confronting a false belief. That is always touchy. She might listen or she might dig in her heels. How she responded would make all the difference in how much improvement in pain and function she would see in the future.

"Listen," I began gently. "If physical therapy made you hurt but your home exercises do not, perhaps you aren't really doing the same stretches or doing them to the extent that the professionals were doing. You have not improved your range of motion with your own program, gradually losing function of your shoulder until you can hardly use it at all. The lack of function and pain that has spread to nearby areas of your body is not due directly to your shoulder injury but to disuse."

"It could be worse if I get injured at physical therapy," she countered.

"It doesn't sound like physical therapy broke a bone or tore a tendon," I answered. "You were sore—very sore—which was predictable when you had not been stretching or exercising. Physical therapy is not likely to injure you. Although it is remotely possible to have an injury at the physical therapy office, the weaker and tighter your muscles and tendons get, the more likely they are to be injured in the course of your normal activities at home."

I leaned forward. "No amount of procedures and medications will improve your mobility and stamina without stretching and exercise. You can only get worse."

It was not easy, but I was able to help Ellen see.

Ellen went to physical therapy. It hurt for the first few weeks. She called on the second week, losing her resolve, but I encouraged her to continue. Every week after that, the pain decreased, and her range of motion increased. She was rightfully proud when she returned to my office, able to raise both arms into the air.

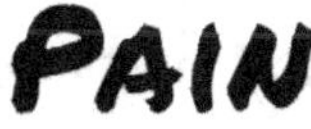

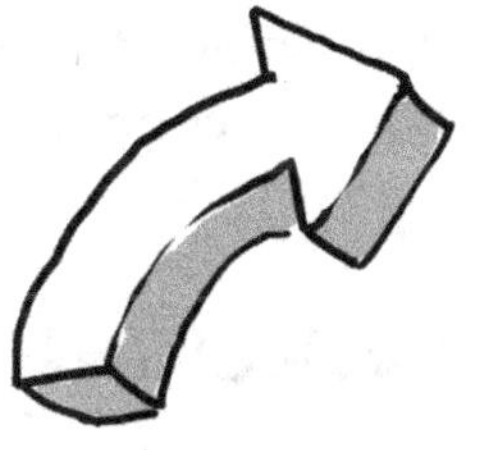

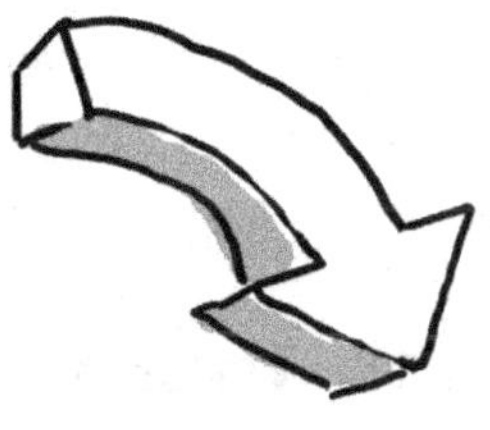

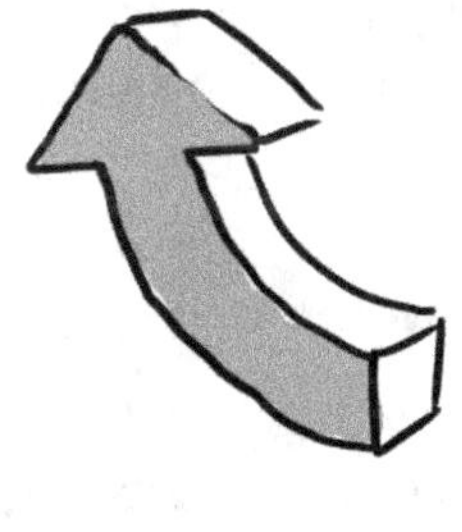

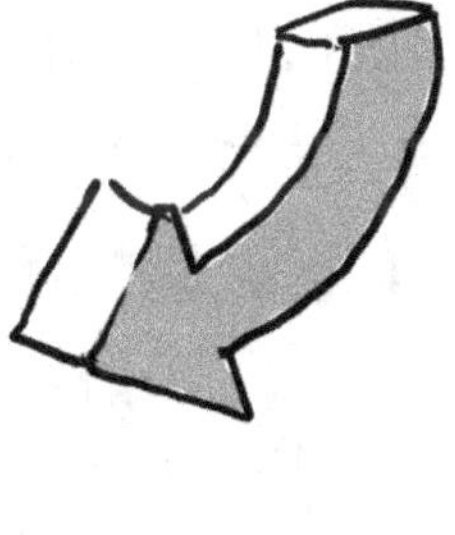

Why Self-made Exercise Programs Don't Work

In my experience, once a patient reaches the point where they have painful limits to their range of motion, effective treatment usually requires physical therapy. The first few weeks of that therapy are going to leave them very sore, not from the original injury or disease but from the surrounding tight, weak muscles that are being stretched. It has to be done though. The key is to start slow and make small increases over time.

Like Ellen, many new patients tell me they are doing regular exercises. When I ask for details about what exercises they are doing and how often, the picture is usually less reassuring. Movements are usually guided by what doesn't cause discomfort and times are inconsistent, usually averaging twice a week or less. It is a rare person who is confident about doing movements that hurt even if they won't cause injury, so homemade exercise programs tend to concentrate on strengths and avoid weaknesses. In cases where there is limited range of motion to a joint or the spine, it may even be impossible for someone to actively move the joint against the pain.

Starting Your Recovery with Physical Therapy

Although it is remotely possible, I've never sent a patient to physical therapy who has come back injured. All of my patients who have gone to all the sessions have improved flexibility, balance, and endurance, and most have had decreased pain. Large studies agree with my experience. Physical therapists are trained to recognize what tendons and muscles need strengthening and stretching and how to do it safely. They will provide a home exercise plan designed specifically for your needs. They can assess your progress and make sure you are doing the movements correctly. They also can do passive stretching to areas of decreased mobility that you cannot actively do on your own.

A Successful Exercise and Stretching Program

A planned exercise program that includes stretching makes an incredible difference in terms of long-term pain control, mobility, and quality of life. To be effective, it must be three things:

- Consistent: Think of exercise as an investment into an account that earns compound interest. You will earn more from doing ten minutes a day than from doing several hours at the end of the week. Once you miss no more than four days of exercise in a month, it may be time to add more time to the sessions. Getting into the habit is the key in the beginning.

- Persistent: You will lose the benefits of exercise even more quickly than you gained them if you slack off. If you have increased pain or have other issues in your life, continue the ten minutes per day at least. Go as slowly as you need, but maintain the habit. Your losses will be much less.

- Structured: You will not get enough of the right kind of exercise if you do not follow a specific program. Day-to-day activities may leave you tired, but your body will subconsciously avoid movements that cause pain. Your job, even if you do manual

I know you will be successful, because you have already shown a desire to address your pain management according to the seven principles outlined in this book. Make it through the first few weeks, and you'll be home free.

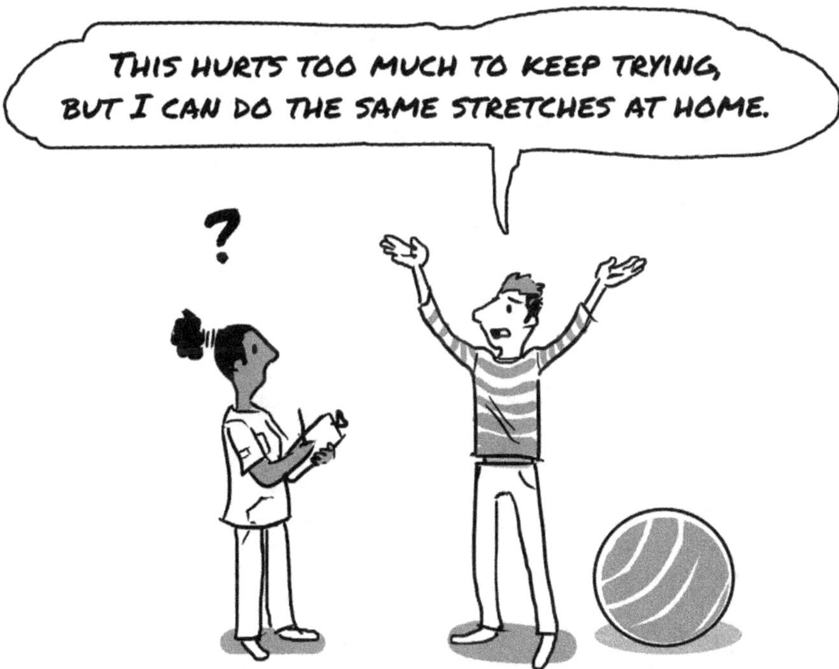

My recommendations:

- Start with a physical therapist. Get a complete assessment and a home exercise plan. If money is a problem, go to two sessions at least. I've told plenty of patients that this is a condition for me to treat them. (I don't make any money off physical therapy.)

- Even better, do a full session of physical therapy to get jump-started on the program. You will be sore, but don't quit. Set a goal for the end of each session with your therapist that you can't achieve on your own. Sometimes I will give a steroid injection to a painful area during the first week a patient is in physical therapy. It often cuts the pain from the new movement in half.

- Go back for reassessment and revision of your program every one to two years or when a new problem arises. Things change, and so will your exercise plan.

The Principle of Conscience

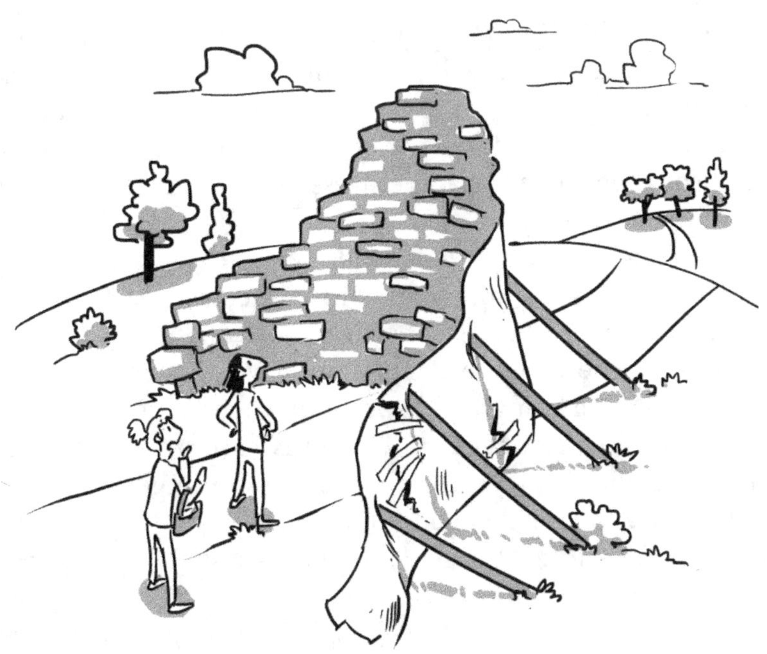

Conscience is a property that must be followed and protected.

Application to pain management: You must often overcome deceptive barriers in your thinking to keep progressing.

Jackie arrived in my office early. She was wearing an athletic warm-up outfit and running shoes.

"I was an athlete in high school and into my mid-twenties," she said. "I had a busy and energetic lifestyle that I loved. In my twenty-sixth year, I began to have increased muscle pain and tenderness after activity. I gave myself more rest and paced my activities, but the pain just got worse."

She began to break down. "One day I found myself crying in pain after climbing two flights of stairs in my apartment building. What made it so much worse is that I had run the four flights of stairs ten times the year before just for exercise."

She continued to pour out her frustration. "I don't understand what's happening or why it hasn't gone away. I can't sleep. When I get stressed, my pain goes through the roof."

I did a full examination, which showed nothing but unusual tenderness throughout her body. I ran blood tests and reviewed her X-rays. Nothing there either.

"Everything adds up to a diagnosis of fibromyalgia," I told her. "I think medical management will help, along with a non-impact exercise program. I would also like you to see a specially trained psychologist."

"This is not in my head!" she cried. "I don't need to see a psychologist. I've always been able to handle stress just fine. It's not my emotions that give out; it's my body."

"Stress affects all of us," I explained. "It increases our perception of pain and causes the same source of pain to increase in intensity. When we reach that critical level of stress, we blow off steam. Some people become angry, some withdraw, and some have physical symptoms. As we develop as human beings, we learn to manage the stress to avoid this critical level. If our personal critical level is high, we don't necessarily need to manage the stress as soon. Chronic pain in general, and fibromyalgia specifically, has changed your critical level. At a point where you used to hardly notice the stress, certainly not enough to get angry, now your body reacts with increased pain. It is a whole new ballgame, and you don't have twenty-six years to spare learning the new rules."

"That's so true," she said. "I've always been the one to be together, the leader. Now I have to hang back. I don't feel I have control anymore."

"That's where the psychologist can help," I replied. "She will help you recognize the new critical level and how to manage it in such a way to minimize your body's reaction to it. You are a successful and reasonable person who has been hit with a devastating illness. Your frustration is normal. The fact that you developed discipline in your life before this illness is a good predictor of your success in overcoming the obstacles it places in your way."

Pain Affects the Whole Person

Most people realize that return to function after a serious illness or injury is affected by both physical and psychological factors. Up to a point, previous coping skills, job satisfaction, and psychological trauma associated with the injury may have a greater impact on recovery than the severity of the injury.

For milder pain, you may already have enough coping skills to meet the challenge without being overwhelmed by anxiety and depression, but everyone has a point where they need help. Do you feel overwhelmed and sad? Psychology is a central pillar in the comprehensive treatment of chronic pain. Trying to overcome the habits and false beliefs that hinder your progress is difficult. Trying to do it when you are in a crisis seems insurmountable. Counselors also help with insomnia, pacing, and establishing treatment goals. One of the most encouraging aspects of psychological treatment is they teach techniques that empower you wherever you are, independent of the counselor.

My recommendations for changing deceptive barriers to your thinking:

- You are a reasonable person who has been hit with a devastating illness. You may need to learn new coping techniques that you didn't need before.

- Use your pain counselor as a sounding board to help you find barriers to victory and as a coach to develop coping skills so that pain doesn't dominate your life.

- For depression and anxiety, the first line treatment is either the option of starting doses of medication or of psychological counseling. The next step is to add the other option. If you still have depression or anxiety symptoms despite medication, or you already are taking two medications, you should add counseling.

6

The Principle of Self-control

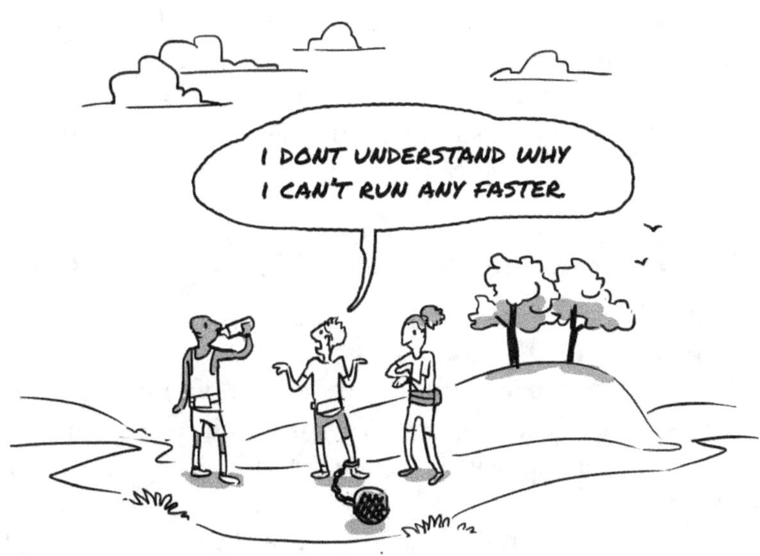

External freedom comes from internal discipline.

Application to pain management: You must control your unhealthy habits to overcome chronic pain.

Bobby's primary-care provider sent him to see me for non-surgical treatments of knee pain. He sat in my office and opened up.

"I have always had a weight problem" he said. "I was overweight as a child and young adult. Now I'm an obese middle-aged man. I've tried diets, but I always went back to eating what I wanted. My parents were both obese, so I've always chalked it up to genetics. That and a coping method for stress."

Bobby laughed ruefully. "I'm a successful businessman. I own a car dealership. Long hours and attention to detail made me successful. Over the last few years though, I've been limited by pain in my knees. I no longer walk out into the lot with my customers. I just sit at my desk in the office. I miss showing the cars to the customers. Even when I take it easy and walk less, my knees still ache by evening despite round-the-clock Ibuprofen.

"What can I do, Doc?" he asked. "I can't walk across the street without pain. I can't walk around the block at all. I saw a knee surgeon who told me I needed knee replacements, but he said I should wait until I can't walk since the implants probably won't last the rest of my life."

I discussed the options with him—injections to the knees to decrease pain and inflammation or a different type of injection that would help cushion the knees. I could deaden the nerves to the knee. "I can also place a small, safe peripheral nerve stimulator on the nerve going to the knee joint that should significantly decrease the pain transmitted from the joint."

Peripheral Nerve Stimulators and Spinal Cord Stimulators

Peripheral nerve stimulators (PNS) use rapid low-voltage fluctuations to interrupt the flow of pain signals along peripheral nerves. A thin wire receiver is placed under the skin, and a removable external unit powers the device. Some of the applications of PNS include pain that continues after surgery to the knee, shoulder, inguinal hernia, and low back.

Spinal cord stimulators (SCS) work the same way as PNS but on the spinal cord's signals to the brain. A thin wire electrode is placed safely in the epidural space and attached outside the spine to a battery that goes under the skin. Some newer devices are rechargeable or have external power units. Spinal cord stimulators are often used to treat "failed back syndrome," a condition where a surgical back fusion fails to stop back pain and radiating pain. They may also be used for certain types of nerve or circulation pain in the limbs.

Bobby was interested in the options. Then I mentioned what, of course, he knew. "You could stop the problem and even give your knees a chance to heal if you lost weight. You might have a much greater battle eating less than I can imagine, but the answer is still exercising more and eating smarter."

He agreed to enter an accountable diet, exercise and weight-loss program. It involved the types of food he ate, as well as fewer calories. In just a week he felt less pain overall, just from eliminating the main suspects in his diet for causing inflammation. He felt excited and continued the plan. Fifty pounds later, he felt a huge difference in his knee pain. Less pain allowed more vigorous exercise, leading to more weight loss. He is still on his way, but he may be able to avoid knee joint replacement after all.

Unhealthy Habits Make Chronic Pain Worse

Healing one part of the body can best be done in a body that is healthy overall. The basics of good health are essential in the treatment of chronic pain. Unhealthy habits like overeating, a sedentary lifestyle, smoking (or vaping), excess alcohol, and/or inappropriate drug use make your pain worse, prevent healing, and compound the problems that limit your life. You cannot wait to deal with these issues until after you get rid of the pain. The unhealthy issues are part of the pain problem.

Treat Bad Habits While Treating Your Pain

Your primary-care doctor is involved in most areas of your general health. For my patients, I reinforce those efforts with education and accountability. I offer a smoking-cessation program that incorporates free counseling and medications, as needed. I also counsel on changes in diet that decrease inflammation, which is known to increase pain. In addition, I advise on supplements and test for deficiencies, and I encourage exercise designed to meet patients' specific needs. I teach my patients to see the treatment of chronic pain as one emphasis in an overall strategy of maintaining good health.

If you can't change your habits even after you know they are hurting you, you may have an addiction. This is common with nicotine, illicit drugs, and overeating. Most people have already learned that those addictions are harmful, but they can't stop the behavior. Addiction can be treated by a specialist, and the barrier can be overcome. Still, a big part of getting rid of unhealthy habits is self-control. Developing self-control in an area of weakness takes a commitment and a system of accountability. It can be done. It has been done. You can live a healthy life.

My recommendations to control your unhealthy habits:

- Stop using nicotine. If you have a nicotine addiction, get in a cessation program to help.

- Get on an exercise program and a controlled diet. Sometimes the last line of defense is at the check-out line. Don't buy unhealthy foods.

- Avoid white or processed flour and sweet foods. Don't use starches to fill up. Limit your alcohol consumption.

The Principle of Character

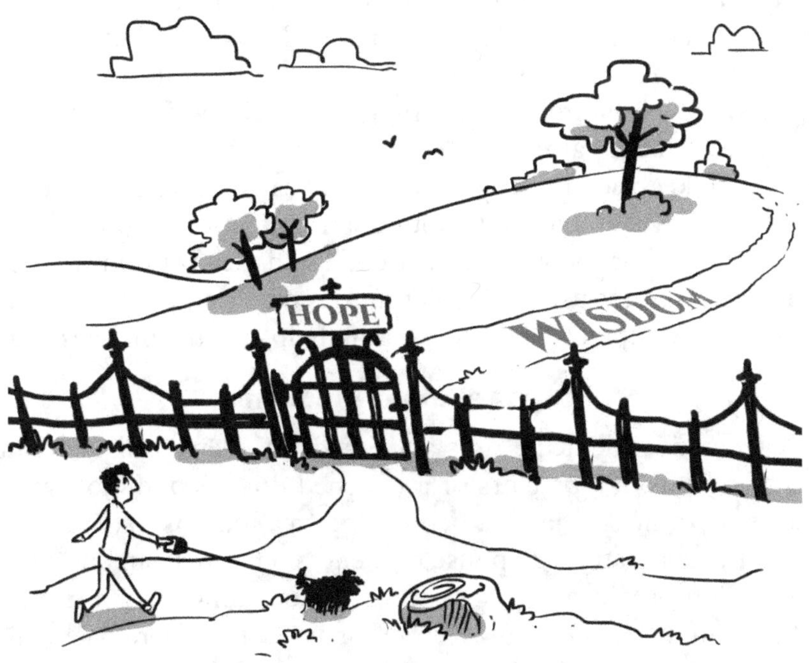

Internal character predicts external success.

Application to pain management: Overcoming chronic pain requires hope for improvement, wisdom about what path to take, and the resilience to keep trying.

have tried everything for this pain in the back of my leg," Janice said as she sat on the examination table, shaking her head. "The pain started after I did a charity fun run, where I had to jump over some boxes set up in a row. The pain was bothersome that day, so I iced the area and took some Ibuprofen.

"I've been athletic all my life, and this wasn't the first time I had pulled a muscle," so I wasn't worried. The problem came when the pain wouldn't go away. Rest didn't help, and over-the-counter medications hardly took the edge off it.

"The pain was aching in one spot high in my leg all the time but sent sharp, streaking pain down the back of my leg when I tried to pick anything up." She teared up. "I'm so frustrated because I have a three-year-old daughter who doesn't understand why Mommy can't hold her.

"After a couple months without progress, I saw my primary-care doctor. He diagnosed me with chronic tendinosis of the hamstring tendon, gave me a corticosteroid injection around the tendon, then got me into physical therapy. I was motivated and saw some improvement with the sharp pain when the tendon was stretched, but the aching pain is still there. It keeps me from sitting too long and aches at night when I want to sleep. My physician told me nothing else could be done, and I would have to live with the pain."

Janice looked me in the eyes. "I was not satisfied with that answer. I decided to seek relief if it can be found. I'm not going to quit."

"I'll review what you've already tried," I said. "The options for helping a tendon in constant use heal faster are pretty slim, but recently a new therapy has developed that does just that: help chronic injuries heal."

Regenerative Medicine

Regenerative medicine uses and injection of live cells or components of cells from a patient's or a matched donor's body to signal injured tissue to heal. The idea behind the treatment is patients do not have a sufficient natural response to mend a tendon, ligament, or joint. The injection provides a catalyst for natural healing, which eliminates most or all of the pain. The most common type of regenerative medicine is platelet-rich plasma (PRP), in which a syringe of blood is withdrawn from the patient and spun down to make platelets more concentrated. Then the platelets are injected into the injured area, causing a cascade healing response to rebuild the tissue. Most insurance companies do not pay for this treatment, but many providers believe this will soon change. In the meantime, the procedure is out of pocket for most patients.

Regenerative medicine, sometimes inaccurately called stem cell therapy, is a new treatment for chronic conditions, especially injured or degenerative joints and tendons. Janice was excited about the potential and delighted that the risks were so low. The one barrier was the price. Her insurance provider, like most, didn't pay for regenerative therapies. However, she and her husband wanted her to take a chance.

I scheduled an appointment to do an injection. After drawing two ounces of blood from her arm, I separated the platelets from the red blood cells using a centrifuge. I was left with a few milliliters of platelet-rich plasma (PRP), which I injected in and around the injured tendon. The PRP was concentrated with healing mediators that signaled her body to hurry its repair. I gave two injections a few weeks apart, combined with a program of physical therapy exercises and daily stretching.

Janice came back for follow-up elated. Within a month she felt less pain, and within a few more she was almost pain free.

"I'm back to running," she told me, "and best of all, I can pick up my daughter again."

The Three Elements of Character

Like Janice, sometimes you can't take no for an answer. You have to keep fighting. The seventh principle to overcome chronic pain provides the key you need to keep going when you feel discouraged, disillusioned, and defeated. Character includes inner strength, but it also means developing the right mindset and the wisdom to use it. Three elements of character are hope for improvement, wisdom to know what to do and how to think, and the inner strength and resilience necessary to walk it out.

Hope requires a positive decision that you will achieve your goal of less pain and greater function. All too often healthcare providers who say nothing more can be done forget to include the first five words of that statement: "As far as I know . . ." Patients walk away thinking they will just have to live with their pain and the limitations it creates. They lose hope. However, pain management is a dynamic field. The last twenty years has seen an explosion of new spinal cord and peripheral nerve stimulators, ablation of small nerves that serve painful joints, and non-surgical relief of spine pain. Hope is your motivator. To face chronic pain, begin by choosing hope.

By reading this book, you have gained a lot of good, practical knowledge regarding the seven principles to overcome chronic pain. Follow these, and you will be using true wisdom when making decisions about your treatment.

To sum them up, begin by getting a pain diagnosis before treatment. Second, use a pain doctor who has broad knowledge of his or her field. Third, don't skip low-risk procedures before moderate- or high-risk procedures. Fourth, push through the pain of the first few weeks of physical therapy, followed by a home exercise program. Fifth, get counseling, if needed, to help you challenge barriers in your thinking that hinder improvement. Sixth, commit to controlling the habits that make your body unhealthy and increase your pain.

The final element of character is resilience—inner toughness. You must keep going. If you quit, you'll get worse. You, not your doctor, your patient representative, or your insurance company must take responsibility for your healing. You might truly have been victimized by trauma or bad genes. There are millions of reasons why you might have disabling chronic pain, but only one person can reach a solution: you. No one else can research and discuss individualized treatment options like you can. No one else can find a team to help you that will agree with your goals and let you retain executive power over your care. You are the one who must keep your medications secure and take them only as agreed. Only you can push past the pain to increase your mobility or work through the barriers that limit your progress. You alone can make the daily decisions that will help you or hurt you.

Some patients get a complete cure—no more chronic pain! Many others continue to have pain, but treatment decreases the pain by 30, 50, or 70 percent or more. The only way to lose is to quit trying. Chronic pain may slow you down. It may make you adjust your plans or lower your expectations or, in a few areas, force you to abandon some goals and replace them with others. Despite that, you can work around restrictions and overcome barriers. In days to come, you will look back and be amazed at how much you enjoy your life, because you have overcome chronic pain.

I'm excited about what lies ahead for you!

What Are the Seven Principles?

n my early twenties, I heard a lecture about how seven biblical principles explained much of history and provided success to those wise enough to live by them. I was a history teacher in a Christian school at the time, so I used the principles in my curriculum.

After many years of medical school, training, and practice, I sought to apply these principles to my medical practice. For years I have shared them with my patients and applied them to their treatment.

The seven principles are components of Wisdom, part of natural law, or basically how things work in the world. Each principle groups many natural laws together, though different people could group them into more or fewer principles depending on their perspective. They are common sense and can be surmised through observation. Few would debate whether they are true; many debate how they are applied, and even more ignore them to their peril.

Some authors have researched the seven principles in depth, though I don't know any who have applied them to pain management. I have not corresponded with any of these authors, but I owe a debt to them for introducing the concepts to me so many years ago. That said, those authors carry no responsibility for any shortcomings in my explanation of the seven principles. My conclusions and any errors that remain are my own.

Glossary

Addiction - a mental illness that prompts a person to use a substance even to their own harm. Since addiction often involves lying about one's use, the addict may, for a time, evade detection.

Adjunctive medications - any pain medication that usually has a different primary indication other than pain. These include antidepressants and anti-epileptics used for nerve pain.

Axial pain - pain in trunk rather than the limbs, most often refers to back and neck pain.

Bulging disk - a beginning stage of herniation. Commonly seen on MRI even in pain-free individuals.

Chronic low back pain - low back pain lasting greater than three months. CLBP is a major source of disability in the USA.

Diagnostic block - local anesthetic placed over a nerve that is either causing pain or transmitting pain from another structure. Elimination of pain indicates that this is the route the pain signals are taking to the brain.

Disability prevention - intense education, physical and occupational therapy, and psychological counseling prevent a slide toward disability, usually in an injured worker.

Disk desiccation - often referred to as a "black disk" because of its appearance on MRI. Dried out internal disk material shrinks over time with age and injury. Such a disk can be pain-free or a source of pain.

Disk extrusion - a protrusion of inner disk material with a stalk-like attachment to the disk.

Disk protrusion - a progressing stage of herniation with length greater than width.

Epidural steroid - placement of steroid solution into the space around the dura (spinal sack) that holds spinal fluid. The steroid soaks through the dura to reach the spinal cord

Facet joint - small joints in the back between vertebrae.

Full-spectrum pain management clinic - a pain clinic that has a comprehensive approach to diagnosis, procedures, medications, and referrals.

Herniated disk - spinal disk that protrudes out from its normal border. When the herniation protrudes towards the spinal cord or an existing spinal root it may cause pain, weakness or numbness in the body.

Lumbar fusion - a moderate risk, extensive spine surgery that fuses the vertebrae together, usually combined with removal of tissue to free up the spinal cord and nerve roots. Most often the fusion is reinforced with hardware (plates, rods and screws).

Medial branch nerve - the nerve that carries pain sensation from the facet joint.

Radiofrequency ablation - high-frequency waves from the tip of a probe cause surrounding tissue to heat up. Targeting the probe on or near a nerve destroys the nerve-conducting tissue without undue damage to surrounding tissue.

MRI - magnetic resonance imaging, uses a magnet rather than x-rays to reveal details of tissues inside the body. Despite its many uses, the MRI provides little help in diagnosing the source in chronic axial spine pain.

Multidisciplinary pain program - pain management immersion program involving medical, psychological, physical medicine, and nursing disciplines for several weeks. Very successful but rare now due to lack of payment.

Myofascial pain - pain coming from muscles or fascia (connective tissue surrounding the muscles) usually producing one or more trigger points.

Neuropathic pain - pain arising from one of the components of the nervous system, such as brain, spinal cord, peripheral nerves or sympathetic nerves. This type of pain may be sharp and electric-like, following the course of the nerve, or may manifest as burning or unpleasant sensations.

Non-impact exercise program - program that avoids jarring and excessive pressure, especially to the joints.

Opioids - compounds derived from or similar to opium that act directly on the opioid receptors in the body to reduce pain.

Pain diagnosis - the specific source and mechanism of pain, as opposed to a radiologic diagnosis which shows structural abnormalities whether they cause pain or not.

Pain psychologist - psychologist with training to treat chronic pain patients. Techniques include relaxation, sleep hygiene, pacing and cognitive therapy.

Peripheral nerve stimulator - a small wire under the skin near a peripheral nerve sends impulses that decrease pain from being transmitted to the brain.

Physical therapy - facilitates movement and strength using tailored stretches and exercises. A home exercise program is best devised by a physical therapist if pain condition is more than mild or areas of the body already have decreased mobility.

Radicular pain - pain caused by direct injury to the nerve root, detected by pain along the nerve root's distribution.

Radiologic diagnosis - diagnosis based on the structural abnormalities seen in imaging. These have little relation to the source of chronic pain, since even pain-free adults usually have many structural abnormalities.

Red flags - signs and symptoms in the spine that warn of the need for emergency surgery stabilization or causes that threaten life or limb.

Referred pain - pain caused by structures other than the nerve root but are interpreted by the brain to be pain coming from areas that share the same nerve root distribution. For example, if a painful facet joint is served by a nerve that returns to the spinal cord through the fifth lumbar spinal root, the brain will think that the pain is in the back, buttock and leg along the area served by the same fifth lumbar spinal root.

Regenerative medicine - placement of active biological healing elements into an area that needs repair. These elements may be platelets, blood cells, placental cells, fat cells, or a mixture of chemicals derived from them.

Sacroiliac joint - joint between the bottom of the spine (sacrum) and the pelvis. Common source of pain in the low back/upper buttocks, especially after pregnancy or years after lower spine fusion surgery.

Second opinion - a commonly used consult to a physician of the same or similar specialty to give advice on treatment plan or diagnosis.

Simple laminectomy/discectomy - a low-risk, usually outpatient spine surgery for true radicular pain, weakness or numbness that removes no or minimal bone.

Spinal cord stimulator - a small wire under the skin along the epidural space sends impulses to the spinal cord that decrease pain from being transmitted to the brain.

Spinal disk - cushioning disk between bony vertebrae in the spine

Transforaminal epidural steroid injection - an epidural injection that is placed with a thin needle through the foramina (exit space for the nerve root).

Translaminar epidural steroid injection - an epidural injection that is placed between the bones in the back of the spine.

Trigger point - tender knots that are a source of radiating pain. Most common location is in the upper back. Trigger points are related to myofascial pain.

True radicular pain - pain arising from inflammation or damage to the nerve root exiting the spine. Most often caused by a herniated disk or overgrowth of bone and ligaments into the spinal canal or foramina (exit space for the nerve root).

Vertebrae - bony part of the spine separated from each other in front by spinal disks and in back by facet joints.

Yellow flags - signs or symptoms in a patient that indicate a barrier to returning to work or normal function.